The Wilderness Expert Long Term Survival Mastery Guide: Expert Techniques for Sustaining Life in the Wild for Extended Periods

Contents

Introduction

Welcome to "The Wilderness Expert Long Term Survival Mastery Guide: Expert Techniques for Sustaining Life in the Wild for Extended Periods." This guide is designed to equip you with the knowledge, skills, and mindset necessary to survive and thrive in the wilderness over long periods. Whether you are an outdoor enthusiast, a seasoned survivalist, or someone seeking to prepare for potential emergencies, this book provides comprehensive insights into long-term wilderness survival.

Purpose of the Guide

The primary aim of this guide is to offer a thorough understanding of the techniques and strategies required for sustained survival in the wild. Unlike short-term survival, which focuses on immediate needs and quick resolutions, long-term survival involves a deeper level of preparation and adaptability. This book delves into the complexities of living off the land for extended periods, ensuring you are well-prepared for any situation that may arise.

The Importance of Long-Term Survival Skills

In today's world, the ability to survive in the wilderness is an invaluable skill set. Natural disasters, unexpected accidents, and unforeseen circumstances can lead to situations where long-term survival knowledge becomes essential. By mastering these skills, you not only increase your chances of survival but also develop a profound connection with nature. Understanding how to live sustainably in the wild fosters a greater appreciation for the environment and enhances your resilience and self-reliance.

How to Use This Book

This guide is structured to provide a logical progression of skills and knowledge, starting with the basics and advancing to more complex techniques. Each chapter builds on the previous ones, creating a cohesive and comprehensive learning experience. Here's how you can get the most out of this book:

1. **Start from the Beginning:** While it might be tempting to jump straight to advanced topics, it is crucial to master the basics

first. Each chapter lays the groundwork for more complex survival skills.

2. **Practice Regularly:** Survival skills are best learned through practice. Whenever possible, apply the techniques discussed in this book in real-life settings. Start with short trips and gradually increase the duration as you become more confident.

3. **Reflect and Adapt:** Survival in the wilderness requires adaptability. Reflect on your experiences and learn from your mistakes. This continuous learning process is essential for long-term success.

4. **Stay Safe:** While practicing survival skills, always prioritize safety. Understand your limits and take necessary precautions to avoid unnecessary risks.

5. **Use the Appendices:** The appendices at the end of the book provide valuable resources, including checklists, resource lists,

and additional reading materials. Use these tools to enhance your learning and preparation.

A Journey into the Wilderness

Embarking on a journey into the wilderness is both a challenge and an adventure. It tests your physical abilities, mental fortitude, and ingenuity. However, with the right knowledge and preparation, it can also be an incredibly rewarding experience. This guide aims to prepare you for that journey, offering you the tools to not only survive but to thrive in the wild.

Final Thoughts

As you delve into the chapters of this book, remember that survival is as much about mindset as it is about skills. Cultivate a positive, resilient attitude, and embrace the learning process. The wilderness can be an unpredictable and demanding environment, but with the right preparation, you can face it with confidence.

Thank you for choosing "The Wilderness Expert Long Term Survival Mastery Guide." May this book be your trusted companion on your journey to mastering long-term wilderness survival.

Chapter 1: Preparing for the Wilderness

Preparing for a long-term wilderness survival situation requires more than just physical readiness; it demands a comprehensive approach that includes mental conditioning, knowledge acquisition, and practical planning. This chapter will guide you through the essential preparatory steps to ensure you are well-equipped for the challenges of the wild.

Essential Mindset and Attitude

Survival in the wilderness is as much about mental strength as it is about physical skills. Cultivating the right mindset is crucial for enduring long-term hardships and remaining resilient in the face of adversity.

1. **Stay Positive:** Maintaining a positive attitude is vital. A hopeful outlook can significantly impact your ability to think clearly and make sound decisions. Practice gratitude, focus on small victories, and remind yourself of your strengths and capabilities.

2. **Embrace Adaptability:** The wilderness is unpredictable, and conditions can change rapidly. Being adaptable means staying flexible in your plans and approaches. Embrace change and be willing to adjust your strategies as needed.

3. **Develop Patience:** Long-term survival often involves waiting—waiting for food, waiting for the weather to improve, waiting for rescue. Cultivating patience helps manage stress and prevents rash decisions.

4. **Mental Toughness:** Build mental toughness through challenges and adversity. Push your limits in controlled environments to understand your physical and psychological boundaries. Practice mindfulness and meditation to enhance your mental resilience.

Physical Conditioning and Fitness

Physical fitness is fundamental to long-term survival. Your body must be capable of enduring strenuous activities, carrying heavy loads, and performing tasks that require strength and stamina.

1. **Cardiovascular Fitness:** Engage in activities that boost your cardiovascular endurance, such as running, hiking, swimming, and cycling. Aim for at least 150 minutes of moderate aerobic activity per week.

2. **Strength Training:** Build muscular strength through exercises like weightlifting, bodyweight exercises (push-ups, pull-ups, squats), and resistance training. Focus on functional movements that mimic survival tasks.

3. **Flexibility and Balance:** Incorporate stretching routines and balance exercises to improve your overall agility and prevent injuries. Yoga and Pilates are excellent practices for enhancing flexibility and balance.

4. **Endurance:** Train for long-duration activities by gradually increasing the length and intensity of your workouts. Participate in long hikes, multi-day treks, or endurance sports to build stamina.

Mental Preparedness and Adaptability

Beyond physical fitness, mental preparedness is essential for effective long-term survival. This involves not only preparing for challenges but also developing the ability to adapt to unforeseen circumstances.

1. **Scenario Planning:** Visualize potential survival scenarios and mentally rehearse your responses. Consider different challenges you might face, such as injuries, extreme weather, or scarcity of resources, and plan how you would handle them.

2. **Stress Management:** Learn techniques for managing stress, such as deep breathing, visualization, and progressive muscle relaxation. Stress can impair your judgment and decision-making abilities, so having tools to manage it is crucial.

3. **Problem-Solving Skills:** Enhance your problem-solving abilities by engaging in activities that require critical thinking and creativity. Puzzles, strategy games, and learning new skills can sharpen your mind and prepare you for the unexpected.

4. **Knowledge Acquisition:** Equip yourself with knowledge about the wilderness and survival techniques. Read books, watch instructional videos, attend survival courses, and practice skills regularly. The more you know, the better prepared you will be to face challenges.

Building a Survival Kit

A well-equipped survival kit is a cornerstone of long-term wilderness survival. It should contain essential items that support your basic needs for shelter, fire, water, and food.

1. **Shelter:** Include a durable tarp, emergency blankets, rope or paracord, and a compact sleeping bag or bivy sack. These items will help you create and maintain a safe, insulated shelter.

2. **Fire:** Pack waterproof matches, a lighter, a ferrocerium rod, and fire-starting tinder such as cotton balls soaked in petroleum jelly. Fire is crucial for warmth, cooking, and signaling for help.

3. **Water:** Carry a water filter, purification tablets, and a durable water container. Staying hydrated is critical, and these tools will help ensure you have access to clean drinking water.

4. **Food:** Include non-perishable, high-energy foods such as energy bars, dried fruits, nuts, and freeze-dried meals. A compact fishing kit and basic trapping supplies can also help you secure food in the wild.

5. **Tools:** Essential tools include a multi-tool, a fixed-blade knife, a folding saw, and a compact shovel. These tools will assist in various tasks, from building shelter to preparing food.

6. **Navigation:** Pack a compass, a detailed map of the area, and a GPS device if possible. Knowing your location and how to navigate the terrain is vital for long-term survival.

7. **First Aid:** A comprehensive first aid kit should contain bandages, antiseptics, pain relievers, tweezers, and any personal medications. Include a first aid manual for reference.

8. **Clothing:** Pack appropriate clothing for the environment, including moisture-wicking layers, a weatherproof jacket, a hat, gloves, and sturdy boots. Layering helps regulate body temperature and protects against the elements.

9. **Communication:** A whistle, signal mirror, and a lightweight emergency radio can help you communicate with rescuers or other survivors.

10. **Miscellaneous:** Include items such as duct tape, sewing kit, insect repellent, sunscreen, and a headlamp with extra batteries. These small items can make a significant difference in your comfort and safety.

Practical Planning

Effective planning is the foundation of successful long-term survival. This involves preparing for your journey, understanding the environment, and having a clear plan for various scenarios.

1. **Research the Area:** Study the geography, climate, flora, and fauna of the area where you plan to survive. Understanding the environment helps you anticipate challenges and identify resources.

2. **Create a Survival Plan:** Outline a detailed survival plan that includes your goals, strategies, and contingency plans. Consider factors such as shelter locations, water sources, food procurement methods, and escape routes.

3. **Practice Skills:** Regularly practice essential survival skills, such as fire starting, shelter building, and navigation. The more proficient you are in these skills, the more confident and prepared you will be.

4. **Emergency Contacts:** Inform a trusted person about your plans, including your location and expected duration. Establish regular check-in times and have a plan for emergency communication.

5. **Physical and Mental Health:** Prioritize your health by maintaining a balanced diet, getting regular exercise, and managing stress. A healthy body and mind are better equipped to handle the rigors of long-term survival.

Chapter 2: Basic Survival Skills

Mastering the basics of survival is essential before delving into advanced techniques. In this chapter, we will cover the fundamental skills necessary for surviving in the wilderness: shelter building, fire starting and maintenance, and water sourcing and purification. These core skills form the foundation of long-term survival and are critical for ensuring your immediate safety and well-being.

Shelter Building Techniques

A well-constructed shelter protects you from the elements, conserves body heat, and provides a safe resting place. Different environments and weather conditions call for different types of shelters.

1. **Understanding Shelter Priorities**

   o **Location:** Choose a safe, dry location away from hazards like falling branches, flash flood zones, and animal trails. Look for natural features that can provide additional protection, such as rock overhangs or dense vegetation.

- ○ **Insulation:** Your shelter must retain heat. Use natural materials like leaves, grass, and pine needles to insulate the interior.

- ○ **Weather Protection:** Ensure your shelter can withstand the prevailing weather conditions. It should be waterproof and wind-resistant.

2. **Types of Shelters**

- ○ **Lean-To:** A simple and effective shelter, especially in wooded areas. Build a frame using sturdy branches and lean additional branches against it at an angle, covering it with leaves, bark, and other debris for insulation.

- ○ **Debris Hut:** Ideal for cold weather. Construct a ridgepole supported by two forked sticks, and pile branches and debris over it to create a thick insulating layer.

- ○ **A-Frame:** Provides excellent rain protection. Build a ridgepole between two trees or supports, then lean branches against both sides, creating an A-shaped structure. Cover with debris for insulation.

- o **Tarp Shelter:** If you have a tarp or emergency blanket, it can be used to create various shelters, such as the A-frame, lean-to, or even a simple tent by tying the corners to trees or stakes.

3. **Building and Maintaining Your Shelter**

- o **Construction:** Start by clearing the ground of sharp objects and debris. Build the frame first, then add layers of insulation and weatherproofing materials.

- o **Maintenance:** Regularly check your shelter for damage, especially after storms. Replace worn or damaged materials as needed to ensure it remains effective.

Fire Starting and Maintenance

Fire is a vital survival tool for warmth, cooking, water purification, and signaling. Knowing how to start and maintain a fire is crucial.

1. **Gathering Materials**

   o **Tinder:** Fine, dry materials that ignite easily, such as dry grass, leaves, bark shavings, and cotton balls. Ensure you have enough tinder to sustain a flame long enough to ignite kindling.

   o **Kindling:** Small sticks and twigs that catch fire from the burning tinder. Collect a variety of sizes, from matchstick thickness to finger thickness.

   o **Fuel:** Larger logs and branches that sustain the fire. Start with smaller pieces and gradually add larger ones as the fire grows stronger.

2. **Fire Starting Techniques**

   o **Using Matches or Lighters:** These are the simplest methods. Shield the flame from wind and rain, light the tinder, and gradually add kindling and fuel.

- Ferrocerium Rod: Scrape the rod with a metal striker to produce sparks. Aim the sparks at the tinder bundle until it ignites.

- Bow Drill: A primitive method that requires a bow, spindle, fireboard, and socket. Rapidly rotate the spindle in the fireboard socket using the bow to create friction and generate an ember. Transfer the ember to a tinder bundle and blow gently until it ignites.

- Flint and Steel: Strike a piece of high-carbon steel against flint to produce sparks. Aim the sparks at the tinder bundle to ignite it.

3. **Maintaining a Fire**

- Fire Lay: Arrange your firewood in a structure that promotes airflow, such as the teepee, lean-to, or log cabin. Proper airflow is essential for sustaining the fire.

- Feeding the Fire: Add fuel gradually, starting with small sticks and progressing to larger logs. Avoid smothering the fire by adding too much fuel at once.

- Extinguishing the Fire: When you no longer need the fire, extinguish it thoroughly by spreading the embers and dousing them with water. Stir the ashes and ensure no embers remain hot.

Water Sourcing and Purification

Securing a reliable source of clean water is paramount for survival. Understanding how to find, collect, and purify water is essential for maintaining hydration and health.

1. **Finding Water Sources**

   - Natural Sources: Look for rivers, streams, lakes, ponds, and springs. Flowing water is generally safer than stagnant water, but all sources should be purified before consumption.

- **Rainwater Collection:** Use tarps, containers, or natural depressions to collect rainwater. Rainwater is generally safe to drink but can be filtered for added safety.

- **Solar Still:** Dig a hole in the ground, place a container in the center, and cover the hole with plastic sheeting. Place a small rock in the center of the plastic to create a low point. Condensation will collect on the plastic and drip into the container.

- **Vegetation:** Some plants, such as vines and cacti, store water. Learn to identify and safely extract water from these plants.

2. **Water Purification Techniques**

- **Boiling:** Bring water to a rolling boil for at least one minute to kill pathogens. This is one of the most reliable methods of purification.

- **Filtration:** Use a commercial water filter or create a homemade filter using layers of sand, charcoal, and gravel to remove impurities. Follow filtration with purification methods to ensure safety.

- **Chemical Purification:** Use water purification tablets or drops, such as iodine or chlorine dioxide. Follow the manufacturer's instructions for proper use.

- **UV Purification:** UV light devices can disinfect water by killing bacteria, viruses, and protozoa. Ensure the water is clear before using UV treatment, as turbidity can reduce effectiveness.

3. **Storing Water**

- **Containers:** Use clean, durable containers for storing purified water. Seal them tightly to prevent contamination.

o **Rotation:** Regularly rotate your water supply to ensure it remains fresh. Store water in a cool, dark place to extend its shelf life.

Practical Exercises

1. **Build a Shelter:** Practice constructing different types of shelters in various environments. Test their durability and comfort under different weather conditions.

2. **Start a Fire:** Experiment with different fire-starting techniques, using natural materials found in your surroundings. Practice maintaining a fire in different weather conditions.

3. **Find and Purify Water:** Locate natural water sources in your area, collect water using different methods, and practice purifying it using boiling, filtration, and chemical treatments.

Chapter 3: Advanced Shelter Construction

In a long-term survival situation, the basic shelter building skills you've learned will need to be expanded upon to create more durable and comfortable living quarters. This chapter delves into advanced shelter construction techniques, focusing on seasonal shelters, insulation and weatherproofing, and long-term shelter maintenance.

Seasonal Shelters

Different seasons require different shelter considerations to ensure safety and comfort. Here, we'll explore the specific needs of summer, winter, and transitional seasons.

1. **Summer Shelters**

   o **Ventilation:** In hot weather, proper ventilation is crucial to avoid overheating. Construct shelters that allow airflow, such as elevated platforms with open sides or A-frame shelters with wide openings.

- **Shade:** Position your shelter to maximize shade, using natural features like trees or creating your own shade with tarps or large leaves.

- **Bug Protection:** Insects can be a significant nuisance and health risk. Use fine mesh netting or tightly woven fabrics to keep insects out of your shelter.

2. **Winter Shelters**

- **Heat Retention:** Insulating your shelter is key to retaining heat. Use natural materials like snow, leaves, and pine boughs to create thick walls and roofing.

- **Snow Shelters:** Quinzee or snow caves can be highly effective. Create a large mound of snow, let it sinter (harden) for a few hours, then hollow it out to create an insulated snow cave.

- **Wind Protection:** Position your shelter to block prevailing winds. Build walls or use natural barriers to shield your shelter from the wind.

3. **Transitional Seasons (Spring and Fall)**

   - **Adaptability:** Build shelters that can be easily modified to accommodate fluctuating temperatures and weather conditions. Consider designs that allow for opening and closing vents or adding and removing insulation.

   - **Rain Protection:** Ensure your shelter is waterproof by using tarps, plastic sheeting, or thick layers of leaves and bark. Create overhangs or drainage trenches to direct water away from your shelter.

Insulation and Weatherproofing

Effective insulation and weatherproofing are critical for creating a comfortable and safe shelter that can withstand the elements over extended periods.

1. **Insulation Materials**

   - **Natural Materials:** Use leaves, grass, pine needles, and moss to insulate your shelter. These materials trap air and provide excellent thermal insulation.

   - **Artificial Materials:** If available, use items like emergency blankets, foam pads, and insulated sleeping bags to enhance your shelter's warmth.

2. **Techniques for Insulation**

   - **Thatch Roofing:** Create a thick thatch roof using layers of grass, reeds, or palm fronds. This provides both insulation and waterproofing.

   - **Double-Wall Construction:** Build a second wall a few inches outside your main shelter wall and fill the gap with insulating materials. This creates a thermal barrier that helps retain heat.

- **Floor Insulation:** Raise your sleeping area off the ground using logs or rocks and cover it with insulating materials to prevent heat loss through conduction.

3. **Weatherproofing Techniques**

   - **Waterproofing:** Use tarps, plastic sheeting, or tightly woven fabrics to create a waterproof barrier over your shelter. Ensure seams are overlapped and secured to prevent leaks.

   - **Windproofing:** Build solid walls using logs, rocks, or tightly packed branches. Seal gaps with mud, clay, or moss to prevent drafts.

   - **Snowproofing:** For winter shelters, pack snow tightly around the exterior to create an insulating and windproof layer.

Long-Term Shelter Maintenance

Maintaining your shelter over the long term is essential to ensure it remains functional and comfortable. Regular maintenance can prevent small issues from becoming major problems.

1. **Routine Inspections**

    o **Structural Integrity:** Check the frame and support structures for signs of wear, rot, or damage. Reinforce or replace weak components as necessary.

    o **Insulation and Weatherproofing:** Inspect insulation materials for signs of compression or moisture buildup. Replace or replenish as needed to maintain effectiveness.

    o **Pest Control:** Regularly check for signs of pests such as insects, rodents, and larger animals. Use natural repellents or traps to keep them at bay.

2. **Seasonal Adjustments**

o **Winter Preparations:** As winter approaches, add extra insulation, reinforce wind barriers, and ensure your shelter is waterproof. Stockpile firewood and other supplies to minimize the need for trips outside in harsh weather.

o **Summer Preparations:** As summer approaches, focus on increasing ventilation, adding shade, and ensuring your shelter remains dry and free of mold.

3. **Repair and Upkeep**

o **Tools and Materials:** Keep essential repair tools and materials on hand, such as a multi-tool, duct tape, cordage, and spare insulation materials.

o **Proactive Repairs:** Address minor issues immediately before they escalate. Regularly tighten bindings, replace worn materials, and clear debris from around your shelter.

Practical Exercises

1. **Build a Seasonal Shelter:** Construct shelters suited for different seasons, practicing the specific techniques and considerations for each. Test their effectiveness in various weather conditions.

2. **Insulate and Weatherproof:** Experiment with different insulation and weatherproofing materials and methods. Create a shelter that is both warm and waterproof, and test its durability over time.

3. **Shelter Maintenance:** Set up a regular maintenance schedule for your shelter. Perform routine inspections, make necessary repairs, and adjust your shelter for seasonal changes.

Chapter 4: Advanced Fire Techniques and Uses

Fire is essential for warmth, cooking, water purification, and signaling for rescue. Beyond basic fire starting, advanced fire techniques and uses can greatly enhance your ability to survive long-term in the wilderness. This chapter covers various fire construction methods, advanced fire-starting techniques, efficient fuel management, and the multiple uses of fire in a survival situation.

Fire Construction Methods

Different fire lays and structures can optimize fire efficiency for various purposes, such as cooking, signaling, or maintaining warmth.

1. **Fire Lays**

   o **Teepee Fire:** Arrange small sticks in a teepee shape with tinder in the center. This structure allows good airflow and is easy to start. It's ideal for quick warmth and boiling water.

- Log Cabin Fire: Stack logs in a square or rectangular shape, creating layers like a log cabin. Place tinder and kindling in the center. This structure burns longer and is great for cooking.

- Star Fire: Arrange larger logs in a star pattern with their ends meeting in the center. As the ends burn, push the logs inward. This fire is efficient for conserving fuel and providing long-lasting heat.

- Dakota Fire Hole: Dig two connected holes in the ground, one for the fire and the other for ventilation. This underground fire is efficient, conceals flames, and reduces smoke, making it ideal for stealth and windy conditions.

2. **Specialty Fires**

- **Reflector Fire:** Build a regular fire with a reflective wall (using logs or rocks) on one side to direct heat toward your shelter. This setup is excellent for warmth and cooking.

- **Long Log Fire:** Lay two long logs parallel to each other with a narrow gap in between. Light a fire in the gap, and as the logs burn, push them together. This fire burns slowly and steadily, providing heat over a long period.

- **Swedish Torch:** Cut a log into sections but keep them connected at the base. Light the center, and the log will burn from the inside out, acting like a stove. This fire is compact, efficient, and great for cooking.

Advanced Fire-Starting Techniques

Mastering multiple fire-starting methods ensures you can always create fire, even in challenging conditions.

1. **Traditional Methods**

- **Fire Plow:** Rub a hard stick back and forth in a groove on a softer wood base. The friction generates heat and creates an ember.

- **Hand Drill:** Twirl a spindle between your hands, pressing it into a fireboard. The friction generates heat and produces an ember. This method requires practice and strong hands.

- **Pump Drill:** Similar to the hand drill but with a weighted flywheel and a string mechanism. Pumping the drill spins the spindle rapidly, making it easier to create an ember.

2. **Modern Methods**

- **Battery and Steel Wool:** Touch steel wool to both terminals of a 9-volt battery. The electrical current will heat the steel wool and create a fire.

- **Magnifying Glass:** Focus sunlight through a magnifying glass onto tinder. The concentrated light can ignite the tinder. This method requires clear skies and dry tinder.

- **Chemical Reactions:** Combine chemicals like potassium permanganate and glycerin to produce an exothermic reaction that generates heat and ignites tinder. Handle chemicals with care and ensure proper storage.

Efficient Fuel Management

Managing your fuel supply effectively is crucial for long-term survival. Understanding how to collect, process, and store fuel can extend your resources significantly.

1. **Collecting Fuel**

   - **Dead and Dry Wood:** Collect dry branches, twigs, and logs from the ground. Avoid green wood as it contains moisture and produces more smoke.

- **Hardwoods vs. Softwoods:** Hardwoods (oak, maple) burn longer and produce more heat, while softwoods (pine, spruce) ignite quickly and burn faster. Use a mix of both for optimal fire management.

2. **Processing Fuel**

   - **Splitting Wood:** Use an axe or knife to split larger logs into smaller pieces. Smaller pieces ignite more easily and burn more efficiently.

   - **Feather Sticks:** Shave a dry stick to create thin curls that catch fire easily. This technique is useful for starting fires in damp conditions.

3. **Storing Fuel**

   - **Keep It Dry:** Store your fuel in a dry, covered area to protect it from rain and moisture. Elevate it off the ground if possible.

- **Stockpile:** Regularly gather and process fuel to maintain a stockpile. This ensures you have a constant supply, especially in adverse weather conditions.

Uses of Fire

Fire is a versatile tool in survival situations. Understanding its various uses can enhance your ability to thrive in the wilderness.

1. **Cooking**

    - **Direct Cooking:** Skewer meat or vegetables on sticks and cook them directly over the flames or coals.

    - **Boiling Water:** Use a pot or canteen to boil water for drinking, cooking, or cleaning. Boiling is one of the most reliable methods to purify water.

    - **Stone Cooking:** Heat flat stones in the fire and use them as a cooking surface. This method distributes heat evenly and reduces the risk of burning food.

2. **Water Purification**

- ○ **Boiling:** Boil water for at least one minute to kill pathogens. In high altitudes, boil for three minutes.

- ○ **Hot Rocks:** Place heated rocks in a container of water to bring it to a boil. This method is useful when you don't have a metal container.

3. **Signaling for Rescue**

- ○ **Smoke Signals:** Create a smoky fire by adding green branches or leaves. Use a blanket or tarp to create puffs of smoke in a specific pattern, such as three short puffs for distress.

- ○ **Signal Fires:** Build multiple fires in a triangular or straight-line pattern to attract attention from rescuers.

4. **Creating Tools**

- ○ **Harden Wooden Tools:** Use fire to harden the tips of wooden tools like spears and digging sticks. Carefully heat the wood, avoiding direct flames, to make it more durable.

- **Char Cloth:** Create char cloth by heating natural fabric in a sealed metal container with a small hole. The fabric will turn into a slow-burning material useful for catching sparks.

5. **Protection**

- **Predator Deterrent:** Fire can deter wild animals from approaching your camp. Keep a fire burning at night for added security.

- **Insect Repellent:** Smoke from a fire can help repel mosquitoes and other insects. Add green vegetation to the fire to create more smoke.

Practical Exercises

1. **Construct Different Fire Lays:** Practice building various fire structures, such as the teepee, log cabin, and Dakota fire hole. Test their effectiveness for cooking, warmth, and signaling.

2. **Experiment with Fire-Starting Methods:** Try traditional and modern fire-starting techniques. Practice under different weather conditions to build confidence and proficiency.

3. **Fuel Management:** Gather, process, and store different types of fuel. Create a stockpile and monitor how different woods burn and how long they last.

4. **Use Fire for Multiple Purposes:** Cook a meal, boil water, signal for rescue, and create tools using fire. Understand the versatility and importance of fire in survival situations.

Chapter 5: Foraging and Hunting for Food

Securing a reliable food source is a fundamental aspect of long-term wilderness survival. In this chapter, we will explore the principles and techniques of foraging and hunting. Understanding edible plants, trapping small game, fishing, and hunting larger animals will provide you with the skills necessary to sustain yourself in the wild.

Edible Plants and Foraging

Foraging for edible plants can provide a consistent and renewable source of nutrition. Identifying safe and nutritious plants is crucial for avoiding potential hazards.

1. **Identifying Edible Plants**

    o **Field Guide:** Carry a comprehensive field guide specific to the region you are in. Familiarize yourself with the most common edible plants and their characteristics.

    o **Universal Edibility Test:** If uncertain, use the Universal Edibility Test. Separate the plant into parts (leaves, stems, roots, etc.), test each part separately, and observe any adverse reactions over 24 hours.

- ○ **Key Identifiers:** Learn to recognize key features of edible plants, such as leaf shape, flower structure, and growth patterns. Common edible plants include dandelions, cattails, clover, and wild garlic.

2. **Harvesting Techniques**

- ○ **Sustainable Foraging:** Only take what you need, and leave enough for the plant to continue growing. Avoid depleting the plant population.

- ○ **Seasonal Considerations:** Understand the seasonal availability of different plants. Some plants are only edible at certain times of the year.

- ○ **Preparation:** Some plants require preparation to remove toxins or improve digestibility. For example, acorns need to be leached to remove tannins.

3. **Common Edible Plants**

- o **Cattails:** Found near water, almost every part of the cattail is edible. The roots, stems, and flower heads can be eaten raw or cooked.

- o **Dandelions:** Leaves, flowers, and roots are edible. Young leaves are less bitter and can be added to salads.

- o **Wild Berries:** Blueberries, blackberries, and raspberries are commonly found in the wild. Ensure proper identification to avoid toxic look-alikes.

- o **Nuts and Seeds:** Acorns, chestnuts, and pine nuts are valuable sources of fats and proteins. Proper preparation is often required.

Trapping and Hunting Small Game

Trapping and hunting small game provide a reliable protein source and require less energy expenditure than hunting larger animals.

1. **Trapping Techniques**

- Snares: Simple wire or cord loops that tighten around the animal when triggered. Set along animal trails or burrow entrances.

- Deadfall Traps: Use a heavy rock or log to crush the animal. The trigger mechanism releases the weight when the animal disturbs it.

- Box Traps: Constructed from natural materials or pre-made, these traps capture animals alive. Bait the trap to attract the target.

2. **Common Traps**

- Figure-4 Deadfall: A simple and effective deadfall trap using three sticks arranged in a figure-4 pattern to support the weight.

- Paiute Deadfall: An improved deadfall trap with a more sensitive trigger mechanism, increasing the chances of success.

- Spring Snare: Uses a bent sapling or branch to add tension, snapping the snare closed quickly when triggered.

3. **Hunting Techniques**

- **Improvised Weapons:** Use makeshift weapons such as spears, slingshots, or bows. Learn to craft and effectively use these tools.

- **Stealth and Patience:** Approach game quietly and from downwind to avoid detection. Patience is key, as sudden movements can scare away the game.

- **Tracking Skills:** Learn to identify animal tracks, scat, and other signs to locate game trails and feeding areas.

4. **Common Small Game**

- **Rabbits and Hares:** Abundant and relatively easy to trap. Look for their burrows and set traps along their trails.

- Squirrels: Found in wooded areas, they can be hunted with slingshots or trapped using snares.

- Birds: Ground-nesting birds and waterfowl can be trapped or hunted. Look for nesting sites and water sources.

Fishing Techniques

Fishing is an excellent way to obtain a reliable food source, especially if you are near a water body. Different techniques can be employed depending on the environment and available resources.

1. **Fishing Methods**

   - Hand Fishing: Also known as noodling, this involves catching fish with your hands. This method requires skill and caution.

   - Spear Fishing: Use a sharpened stick or an improvised spear to catch fish in shallow waters. Patience and accuracy are essential.

- **Fishing Lines and Hooks:** Use improvised or manufactured lines and hooks. Bait the hook with insects, worms, or small fish.

2. **Constructing Fish Traps**

- **Weirs and Fences:** Build barriers in streams or rivers to guide fish into a trap. Use rocks or sticks to construct the barriers.

- **Basket Traps:** Weave a basket with a funnel entrance. Fish swim in but cannot find their way out. Place the trap in a stream or along a shoreline.

3. **Preserving Fish**

- **Drying:** Clean and fillet the fish, then hang them in the sun to dry. This method requires low humidity and adequate airflow.

- **Smoking:** Build a smoker using a simple frame covered with a tarp or other material. Smoke the fish over a low fire for several hours.

- **Salting:** Cover the fish in salt and let it cure for several days. Salt draws out moisture and prevents bacterial growth.

Hunting Larger Game

Hunting larger game requires more skill, energy, and resources but provides a significant food supply. Understanding tracking, stalking, and proper use of weapons is essential.

1. **Tracking Larger Game**

   - **Identifying Tracks:** Learn to identify the tracks of common large game animals such as deer, elk, and wild boar. Note the size, shape, and gait patterns.

- ○ **Scat and Sign:** Look for scat, broken branches, and other signs of animal activity. This helps determine recent presence and behavior.

- ○ **Water Sources:** Large game frequently visits water sources. Set up ambush points or follow tracks to these areas.

2. **Stalking and Ambushing**

- ○ **Stealth Techniques:** Move slowly and quietly, using natural cover to hide your approach. Pay attention to wind direction to avoid alerting animals with your scent.

- ○ **Ambush Points:** Set up near feeding areas, trails, or water sources. Remain patient and still, waiting for the game to come within range.

- ○ **Shooting Accuracy:** Practice with your chosen weapon to ensure accuracy. Proper shot placement is crucial for a quick, humane kill.

3. **Processing and Preserving Meat**

   - **Field Dressing:** Quickly and efficiently remove the animal's internal organs to prevent spoilage. Use a sharp knife and follow proper techniques to avoid contaminating the meat.

   - **Butchering:** Cut the meat into manageable pieces. Remove bones and fat to reduce weight and improve storage.

   - **Preservation Methods:** Dry, smoke, or salt the meat to preserve it. These methods prevent bacterial growth and extend the shelf life of the meat.

Practical Exercises

1. **Foraging Practice:** Spend time in different environments identifying and collecting edible plants. Test your knowledge and practice sustainable harvesting techniques.

2. **Trap Setting:** Build and set various traps for small game. Monitor their effectiveness and make adjustments as needed.

3. **Fishing Techniques:** Practice different fishing methods, including hand fishing, spear fishing, and using lines and hooks. Construct fish traps and test their effectiveness.

4. **Hunting Skills:** Develop tracking, stalking, and shooting skills for hunting larger game. Practice field dressing and butchering techniques.

Chapter 6: Water Procurement and Purification

Water is essential for survival, more so than food. Securing a reliable and safe water source is critical in long-term wilderness survival. In this chapter, we'll explore various methods for finding, collecting, and purifying water to ensure it is safe to drink.

Finding Water Sources

Understanding where and how to find water is the first step in securing this vital resource.

1. **Natural Water Sources**

   - **Rivers and Streams:** Flowing water is typically safer to drink than stagnant water. Look for clear, running water, and follow it upstream to find cleaner sources.

   - **Lakes and Ponds:** These can be good sources but often require purification due to stagnant conditions that can harbor bacteria and parasites.

o **Springs:** Natural springs are one of the safest water sources, as they often emerge from underground, filtered through layers of rock and soil.

2. **Indicators of Water**

  o **Vegetation:** Lush, green vegetation often indicates a nearby water source. Plants like willows and cottonwoods typically grow near water.

  o **Animal Trails:** Wildlife often follows trails that lead to water sources. Observe the direction of animal tracks.

  o **Terrain:** Water tends to collect in low-lying areas. Look for depressions, valleys, or natural basins where water might accumulate.

  o **Morning Dew:** Collecting dew from plants in the early morning can provide small amounts of water.

3. **Improvise Water Sources**

- o **Solar Still:** Dig a hole, place a container in the center, and cover the hole with a plastic sheet. Place a small rock in the center of the sheet to create a dip, and the sun will evaporate moisture from the ground, condensing on the plastic and dripping into the container.

- o **Transpiration Bags:** Tie a clear plastic bag around a leafy branch. The plant will release moisture into the bag through transpiration, collecting water droplets.

Collecting Water

Effective methods for collecting water can maximize your supply and ensure it remains uncontaminated.

1. **Direct Collection**

   - o **Containers:** Always carry containers such as bottles, canteens, or collapsible bladders for water collection.

- **Improvised Containers:** Use items like tree bark, large leaves, or even a shirt to collect and transport water if no containers are available.

2. **Rainwater Collection**

   - **Rain Catchment System:** Set up a tarp or large piece of plastic to funnel rainwater into a container. Ensure the catchment area is clean to avoid contamination.

   - **Natural Basins:** Look for natural rock basins or depressions that collect rainwater. These can provide significant amounts of water during rainfall.

Water Purification

Purifying water is essential to remove harmful pathogens and contaminants that can cause illness.

1. **Boiling**

- **Boiling Water:** Boil water for at least one minute to kill bacteria, viruses, and parasites. At higher altitudes, boil for three minutes.

- **Improvised Boiling:** Use heated rocks placed in a container of water if you don't have a metal pot. Ensure the container is heatproof.

2. Filtration

- **Commercial Filters:** Portable water filters can remove most bacteria and protozoa. Choose filters with a pore size of 0.1 microns or smaller for the best results.

- **DIY Filtration:** Create a simple filter using layers of sand, charcoal, and gravel in a container with a small hole at the bottom. Pour water through this filter to remove large particles and some pathogens.

3. Chemical Purification

- **Water Purification Tablets:** Follow the instructions on the package. These tablets typically use iodine or chlorine to disinfect water.

- **Household Bleach:** Add two drops of unscented household bleach per quart/liter of water. Let it stand for 30 minutes before drinking.

4. **UV Purification**

- **UV Light:** UV purifiers use ultraviolet light to kill pathogens. These devices are portable and effective but require batteries or solar charging.

- **Solar Disinfection (SODIS):** Fill clear plastic bottles with water and leave them in direct sunlight for at least six hours. The UV rays from the sun will kill many harmful microorganisms.

5. **Natural Methods**

- Charcoal: Use charcoal from your fire to create a rudimentary filter. Crush the charcoal and use it in a layered filter system.

- Plants: Some plants, such as certain types of reeds and water lilies, can help filter water. Be cautious and knowledgeable about which plants to use.

Storing Water

Proper storage techniques can prevent contamination and ensure your water supply remains safe.

1. **Clean Containers**

   - Sterilize Containers: Clean and sterilize containers before use. Boil them or use a bleach solution to kill any pathogens.

   - Sealed Containers: Use containers with tight-fitting lids to prevent contamination from dirt, insects, or other debris.

2. **Avoiding Contamination**

   o **Separate Drinking and Washing Water:** Use separate containers for drinking water and water used for washing or cooking to avoid cross-contamination.

   o **Store in Cool, Dark Places:** Keep water containers out of direct sunlight to prevent the growth of algae and bacteria.

3. **Rotating Water Supplies**

   o **Regular Rotation:** If storing water long-term, rotate your supply regularly to ensure freshness. Mark containers with the date of collection.

   o **Monitoring Quality:** Check stored water periodically for any signs of contamination or spoilage, such as cloudiness, odor, or taste changes.

Practical Exercises

1. **Locate and Collect Water:** Practice finding natural water sources in different terrains. Use vegetation, animal trails, and terrain features as guides.

2. **Build a Solar Still:** Construct a solar still using basic materials and observe the water collection process.

3. **Purify Water:** Experiment with different water purification methods, such as boiling, filtration, and chemical treatment. Compare the effectiveness and ease of each method.

4. **DIY Filters:** Create a DIY water filter using natural materials and test its effectiveness by filtering muddy or cloudy water.

5. **Store Water:** Practice proper storage techniques, including sterilizing containers and monitoring stored water for contamination.

Chapter 7: Shelter Building and Maintenance

A well-constructed shelter is essential for protection from the elements and maintaining body heat, critical factors in long-term wilderness survival. In this chapter, we will explore various shelter types, construction techniques, and maintenance strategies to ensure comfort and safety in the wild.

Importance of Shelter

Shelter serves multiple purposes beyond mere protection from weather:

1. **Protection from Elements:** Shields from rain, wind, snow, and excessive sun exposure.

2. **Preservation of Body Heat:** Helps regulate body temperature, preventing hypothermia and heat-related illnesses.

3. **Psychological Comfort:** Provides a sense of security and peace of mind, crucial for mental well-being in survival situations.

Shelter Types

Choosing the right type of shelter depends on factors such as location, weather conditions, available materials, and personal preference.

1. **Natural Shelters**

   ○ **Caves and Rock Overhangs:** Ready-made shelters offering excellent protection from the elements. Ensure safety from wildlife and falling debris.

   ○ **Large Trees:** Utilize large, sturdy trees with dense foliage for natural cover. Build platforms or lean-tos against the tree trunk.

2. **Improvised Shelters**

   ○ **Lean-to:** Construct a simple shelter using a ridgepole leaning against a support (tree, rock, or other vertical structure). Cover the roof with leaves, branches, or a tarp.

- A-frame Shelter: Similar to a lean-to but with a ridgepole supported by two vertical poles, forming an 'A' shape. Offers better rain runoff.

- **Debris Hut:** Frame made from sturdy branches and covered with a thick layer of leaves, grass, or other debris. Provides insulation and wind protection.

3. **Tarp Shelters**

- **Tarp Lean-to:** Use a lightweight tarp or poncho as the main shelter material. Attach one edge to a ridge line and stake out the other corners.

- **Tarp A-frame:** Create an 'A' frame using a tarp stretched between two trees or poles. Stake down the sides for stability.

Shelter Construction Techniques

Building a sturdy and effective shelter requires careful planning and execution to ensure durability and comfort.

1. **Site Selection**

   o **Flat Ground:** Choose a level area free from rocks, roots, and potential water runoff.

   o **Natural Features:** Utilize natural windbreaks, such as large rocks or dense vegetation.

   o **Drainage:** Avoid low-lying areas prone to flooding. Ensure proper water runoff around the shelter.

2. **Framework**

   o **Support Structures:** Use sturdy materials for support poles, such as saplings, fallen branches, or trekking poles.

   o **Lashing:** Secure poles together using natural cordage (vines, roots) or improvised materials (paracord, shoelaces).

3. **Insulation and Covering**

- **Debris:** Layer leaves, grass, ferns, or pine needles to create a thick insulation layer on top of the shelter.

- **Waterproofing:** Use tarps, ponchos, or large leaves to cover the roof and sides. Ensure overlapping layers to prevent water penetration.

4. **Ventilation**

- **Airflow:** Leave gaps or vents near the base or top of the shelter to allow for airflow. This prevents condensation buildup and improves comfort.

Shelter Maintenance

Maintaining your shelter ensures it remains effective and comfortable throughout your stay in the wilderness.

1. **Regular Inspections**

- **Check Structure:** Inspect support poles, lashings, and roofing materials for signs of wear or damage.

- o **Repair:** Reinforce weak spots, replace damaged materials, and adjust for changes in weather conditions.

2. **Weather Adaptation**

   - o **Snow and Ice:** Remove snow buildup from the roof to prevent collapse. Reinforce with additional insulation against cold.

   - o **Rain and Wind:** Secure tarps and tighten lashings to prevent leaks and ensure stability in windy conditions.

3. **Wildlife and Pests**

   - o **Animal Proofing:** Use odor deterrents or secure food away from the shelter to prevent wildlife from approaching.

   - o **Insect Control:** Use mosquito nets, repellents, or smoke from a fire to deter insects from entering your shelter.

4. **Fire Safety**

- **Distance:** Position your shelter a safe distance from your fire pit to prevent accidental fires or smoke damage.

- **Spark Arrestors:** Use rocks or metal sheets around the fire to contain sparks and prevent them from reaching the shelter.

Practical Exercises

1. **Build Different Shelter Types:** Practice constructing lean-tos, A-frames, and debris huts using available materials in different environments.

2. **Night Stay:** Spend a night in each shelter type to evaluate comfort, warmth, and protection from weather conditions.

3. **Maintenance Drills:** Regularly inspect and maintain your shelters during extended stays in the wilderness. Practice quick repairs and adjustments.

4. **Emergency Shelters:** Learn to build emergency shelters quickly using minimal materials, such as a poncho or emergency blanket.

Chapter 8: Firecraft and Fire Management

Fire is a versatile tool in wilderness survival, providing warmth, cooking capabilities, light, protection, and signaling. In this chapter, we will delve into the essential skills of firecraft, including fire starting methods, fire management, and safe practices to ensure fire serves as a reliable asset in your survival toolkit.

Importance of Fire

Fire serves multiple critical functions in wilderness survival:

1. **Heat and Warmth:** Provides warmth in cold environments, preventing hypothermia and maintaining body temperature.

2. **Cooking and Purification:** Allows for cooking food, boiling water to purify it, and making hot drinks for hydration.

3. **Light and Visibility:** Illuminates surroundings at night, aiding in tasks, navigation, and signaling for rescue.

4. **Psychological Comfort:** Boosts morale and provides a sense of security and normalcy in a challenging environment.

Fire Starting Methods

Mastering various fire starting techniques ensures you can ignite a fire under different conditions and with minimal resources.

1. **Primitive Methods**

   o **Friction Fire:** Use a bow drill or hand drill to generate friction between two pieces of wood, creating an ember. Requires practice and suitable materials.

   o **Fire Plow:** Rub a hardwood stick against a softer wood base to create friction and generate an ember.

   o **Flint and Steel:** Strike a piece of flint or quartz with a steel striker to create sparks that ignite char cloth or a tinder bundle.

2. **Modern Methods**

   o **Lighters and Matches:** Carry waterproof matches or a butane lighter as reliable, quick fire starters. Ensure to keep them dry.

- **Fire Steel:** Use a ferrocerium rod (fire steel) and striker to produce sparks that ignite tinder. Effective in wet conditions.

3. **Chemical Ignition**

- **Fire Starters:** Commercial fire starter blocks, cubes, or gels can ignite even in adverse weather conditions. Carry these as backups.

Tinder and Fire Lays

Preparing and arranging materials properly is crucial for successful fire ignition and maintenance.

1. **Tinder Materials**

- **Natural Tinder:** Dry leaves, grass, bark shavings, and pine needles are readily available and easily ignited.

- **Processed Tinder:** Cotton balls coated with petroleum jelly, char cloth, or lint from clothing make excellent fire starters.

2. **Fire Lays**

   o **Teepee Fire Lay:** Arrange tinder in a cone shape with kindling leaned against it. This structure allows for good airflow and quick ignition.

   o **Log Cabin Fire Lay:** Build a square structure with larger logs or branches, leaving a space in the center for tinder and kindling. Provides a long-lasting fire once established.

   o **Lean-to Fire Lay:** Place kindling against a large log or rock, creating a sheltered space for tinder. This structure protects the fire from wind and rain.

Fire Management and Safety

Maintaining control over your fire is crucial for safety and efficient use of resources.

1. **Fire Site Selection**

   o **Clearance:** Clear the area around your fire site of dry grass, leaves, and other flammable materials.

- **Ventilation:** Ensure your fire is not located under overhanging branches or near flammable structures. Allow for proper airflow.

2. **Building and Controlling Flames**

   - **Start Small:** Begin with a small fire using tinder and kindling. Gradually add larger fuel pieces to build a sustainable flame.

   - **Fire Size:** Adjust the size of your fire based on your needs—larger fires for warmth and cooking, smaller fires for light and signaling.

   - **Fuel Management:** Collect and prepare additional fuel before starting the fire to maintain a steady heat source.

3. **Extinguishing and Safety**

   - **Water Method:** Pour water over the fire, stirring with a stick to ensure all embers are extinguished.

- **Dirt Method:** Cover the fire with dirt, sand, or ashes. Stir and mix thoroughly to smother any remaining embers.

- **Monitor and Secure:** Ensure the fire is completely out before leaving the site. Feel for heat with the back of your hand to confirm extinguishment.

Fire for Survival Situations

Understanding strategic uses of fire in survival scenarios enhances your overall preparedness.

1. **Signaling for Rescue**

   - **Smoke Signals:** Generate thick smoke by adding green vegetation or damp materials to your fire. Create three smoke signals in quick succession as a distress signal.

   - **Flare and Light Signals:** Use the intensity and rhythm of your fire's light to signal for help at night.

2. **Long-Term Fire Maintenance**

- **Sustaining Fire:** Learn techniques for maintaining a fire over extended periods, such as banking coals and feeding consistent fuel.

- **Night Fires:** Keep a small fire burning at night for warmth and protection, adding fuel as needed to maintain a steady flame.

Practical Exercises

1. **Fire Starting Practice:** Experiment with different fire starting methods in varying weather conditions (dry, wet, windy).

2. **Tinder Collection:** Identify and gather natural tinder materials from your surroundings. Test their effectiveness in starting fires.

3. **Fire Lay Construction:** Build teepee, log cabin, and lean-to fire lays. Compare their efficiency and sustainability.

4. **Night Fire Management:** Practice maintaining a fire throughout the night, learning to bank coals and adjust fuel as needed.

Chapter 9: Navigation and Orienteering

Navigation skills are crucial for wilderness survival, allowing you to find your way, avoid getting lost, and reach safety or civilization. In this chapter, we will explore essential navigation techniques, tools, and strategies to help you confidently navigate through diverse wilderness environments.

Importance of Navigation

Understanding navigation is vital for several reasons:

1. **Preventing Getting Lost:** Helps maintain situational awareness and ensures you can return to camp or find your way out of unfamiliar terrain.

2. **Finding Resources:** Allows you to locate water sources, food, and shelter based on maps and environmental cues.

3. **Safety and Rescue:** Enables you to communicate your location accurately in case of emergency and increases your chances of being found.

Basic Navigation Tools

Mastering the use of essential navigation tools enhances your ability to navigate effectively.

1. **Map and Compass**

   ○ **Topographic Map:** Study contour lines, terrain features, water sources, and landmarks to understand the landscape.

   ○ **Compass:** Learn to take bearings, orient the map, and follow a chosen direction using a magnetic compass or orienteering compass.

2. **GPS (Global Positioning System)**

   ○ **Handheld GPS Device:** Provides accurate coordinates, tracks your movement, and marks waypoints for navigation. Ensure it is properly charged and has updated maps.

3. **Natural Navigation**

- **Sun:** Use the position of the sun to determine direction—east in the morning, west in the afternoon.

- **Stars:** Use constellations such as the North Star (Polaris) to find north at night.

- **Landmarks:** Recognize natural landmarks like mountains, rivers, and distinctive trees for orientation.

Orienteering Skills

Orienteering involves navigating from point to point using only a map, compass, and environmental clues.

1. **Map Reading Skills**

   - **Orientation:** Align the map with the surrounding terrain using a compass to match north on the map with magnetic north.

   - **Scale and Distance:** Estimate distances using the map's scale. Use features like contour lines to understand elevation changes.

2. **Compass Use**

   ○ **Taking Bearings:** Use the compass to determine your current direction or a desired direction to navigate towards a specific point.

   ○ **Following a Bearing:** Keep the compass level and steady to maintain accuracy. Periodically check your bearing as you navigate.

3. **Route Planning**

   ○ **Choosing a Route:** Select the safest and most efficient path based on terrain, obstacles, and available resources.

   ○ **Waypoints:** Mark key waypoints along your route for reference. Use prominent features that are easy to identify.

Navigation Techniques

Practice these techniques to enhance your navigation proficiency in wilderness settings.

1. **Dead Reckoning**

   - **Pace Count:** Estimate distance traveled by counting steps. Adjust for terrain and pace to maintain accuracy.

   - **Handrails:** Follow natural features like rivers or ridges that act as guides along your route.

2. **Aiming Off**

   - **Offset Navigation:** Adjust your route slightly to one side of your target point. This ensures you reach your destination even if you miss directly.

3. **Back Bearing**

   - **Reverse Compass Direction:** Take a bearing from your current location back to a known point. Use this to confirm your position or backtrack if needed.

Survival Navigation Tips

In emergency situations, adapt your navigation strategies to prioritize safety and swift resolution.

1. **Stay Put:** If lost, stay calm and assess your surroundings. Use signaling techniques to alert rescuers to your location.

2. **Build a Signal Fire:** Create a smoke signal during the day or a bright flame at night to attract attention.

3. **Create Shelter:** Construct a visible shelter or use natural formations to stay protected while awaiting rescue.

Practical Exercises

1. **Map Reading:** Practice interpreting topographic maps and identifying key terrain features.

2. **Compass Skills:** Conduct exercises in taking bearings, orienting maps, and navigating towards waypoints.

3. **Night Navigation:** Experiment with navigating at night using natural navigation cues like stars and landmarks.

4. **Orienteering Courses:** Participate in orienteering courses or create your own routes to practice navigation under pressure.

Chapter 10: Food Procurement in the Wilderness

Survival in the wilderness requires securing adequate nutrition to sustain energy levels and maintain health. This chapter focuses on essential techniques and strategies for procuring food from the natural environment, ensuring you can sustain yourself during extended stays or emergencies.

Importance of Food Procurement

Understanding how to find, catch, and prepare food in the wild is crucial for several reasons:

1. **Energy and Nutrition:** Provides essential nutrients, calories, and hydration to maintain physical and mental capabilities.

2. **Long-Term Sustainability:** Enables prolonged survival by supplementing stored rations or emergency supplies.

3. **Mental Well-Being:** Boosts morale and provides a sense of accomplishment and connection with the natural environment.

Foraging for Wild Edibles

Identifying and safely harvesting edible plants and fungi can supplement your diet with valuable nutrients and calories.

1. **Edible Plant Identification**

   - **Research:** Study local flora guides or attend wilderness survival courses to learn to identify edible plants, berries, nuts, and roots.

   - **Universal Edibility Test:** Conduct a safety test by touching, smelling, and tasting small portions of a plant to confirm its edibility.

2. **Common Edible Plants**

   - **Wild Berries:** Look for familiar berries like blueberries, raspberries, and blackberries. Avoid berries with a bitter or soapy taste.

- **Edible Greens:** Identify and gather edible leaves, shoots, and roots such as dandelion greens, wild onions, and cattail roots.

- **Nuts and Seeds:** Harvest and consume nuts like acorns, pine nuts, and sunflower seeds after proper processing to remove bitterness or toxins.

3. **Safe Foraging Practices**

- **Avoid Toxic Plants:** Know which plants are poisonous and avoid them. Pay attention to look-alike species that may be harmful.

- **Harvest Sustainably:** Gather only what you need and leave enough for wildlife and future growth.

Hunting and Trapping

Learning effective techniques for hunting and trapping wild game can provide a sustainable protein source in survival situations.

1. **Basic Hunting Skills**

- Tracking: Learn to identify animal tracks, droppings, and signs of feeding to locate potential game trails.

- Quiet Movement: Practice stealth and patience when stalking prey. Avoid sudden movements and excessive noise that could startle animals.

2. **Improvised Weapons and Tools**

- Spear: Create a spear using a sturdy stick and a sharp object like a knife or stone. Use for fishing or hunting small game.

- Snares and Traps: Construct simple traps using natural materials to capture small mammals or birds. Ensure traps are legal and humane.

3. **Fishing Techniques**

- Handline or Fishing Pole: Use improvised or basic fishing gear to catch fish from rivers, lakes, or streams.

- **Primitive Fishing Methods:** Learn to fashion fishhooks from bone or thorns. Use natural bait or improvised lures.

Water-Based Food Sources

Exploit aquatic resources for additional food options in wilderness environments.

1. **Shellfish and Crustaceans**

   - **Mollusks:** Harvest clams, mussels, and snails from tidal zones or freshwater sources. Cook thoroughly to avoid food poisoning.

   - **Crayfish and Crabs:** Use traps or hand capture methods to gather freshwater crayfish or coastal crabs.

2. **Aquatic Plants and Algae**

   - **Edible Seaweeds:** Identify and safely harvest edible seaweeds rich in vitamins and minerals from coastal areas.

- **Water Lilies and Bulrushes:** Gather and prepare aquatic plants found in ponds, lakes, and slow-moving streams.

Preparation and Cooking

Proper preparation and cooking methods ensure safety and maximize nutritional value from wild foods.

1. **Cleaning and Processing**

   - **Gutting and Skinning:** Prepare animals and fish by removing internal organs and skin. Ensure thorough cleaning to prevent contamination.

   - **Filleting and Deboning:** Use sharp knives to fillet fish or remove bones from small game for easier cooking.

2. **Cooking Techniques**

   - **Roasting and Grilling:** Cook meat and fish over an open flame or hot coals on a spit or improvised grill.

   - **Boiling and Stewing:** Use a pot or container to boil water and cook ingredients together to make soups or stews.

- **Smoking and Drying:** Preserve meat and fish by smoking over a low fire or sun-drying to extend shelf life.

3. **Edible Parts and Preservation**

  - **Edible Insects:** Consider insects as a protein source. Collect and cook insects like grasshoppers, ants, and beetle larvae.

  - **Food Preservation:** Dry excess food in the sun or smoke to store for future consumption. Use natural preservatives like salt or vinegar where available.

Practical Exercises

1. **Foraging Excursions:** Identify and gather edible plants and berries from local environments. Record observations and confirm identifications.

2. **Hunting Simulations:** Practice stalking and tracking exercises to understand wildlife behavior and improve hunting skills.

3. **Fishing Trips:** Test fishing techniques using improvised or basic fishing gear. Experiment with different baits and fishing locations.

4. **Food Preparation:** Cook and taste-test wild foods using various cooking methods. Evaluate nutritional content and palatability.

Chapter 11: Water Sourcing and Purification

Water is essential for survival, making it crucial to know how to find, collect, and purify water in the wilderness. This chapter covers essential techniques, tools, and strategies for ensuring safe hydration in diverse wilderness environments.

Importance of Water

Understanding water sourcing and purification is vital for several reasons:

1. **Hydration:** Maintains bodily functions, regulates body temperature, and prevents dehydration.

2. **Health and Safety:** Ensures water is free from harmful contaminants and pathogens.

3. **Long-Term Survival:** Provides access to clean water for drinking, cooking, and sanitation needs.

Finding Water Sources

Identifying and locating reliable water sources in the wilderness is the first step to ensuring hydration.

1. **Natural Water Sources**

   ○ **Rivers, Streams, and Creeks:** Look for flowing water that is less likely to be stagnant or contaminated.

   ○ **Lakes and Ponds:** Collect water from still bodies of water, preferably away from shorelines where contaminants may accumulate.

   ○ **Natural Springs:** Locate and assess spring water for purity and availability.

2. **Rainwater Collection**

   ○ **Rainwater Catchment:** Use tarps, ponchos, or natural depressions to collect rainwater during precipitation events.

○ **Containers:** Carry collapsible or lightweight containers for storing collected rainwater.

3. **Morning Dew and Vegetation**

○ **Dew Collection:** Use absorbent materials like cloth or vegetation to collect dew from plants early in the morning.

○ **Plant Transpiration:** Tie a plastic bag around leafy branches to collect water evaporating from the leaves.

Water Purification Methods

Ensuring water is safe for consumption involves treating and purifying collected water from natural sources.

1. **Boiling**

○ **Boil Water:** Bring water to a rolling boil for at least 1 minute (3 minutes at higher altitudes) to kill harmful bacteria, parasites, and viruses.

- **Cooling:** Allow boiled water to cool before drinking or storing.

2. **Filtration**

   - **Portable Filters:** Use portable water filters or purifiers designed to remove bacteria, protozoa, and sediment from untreated water.

   - **DIY Filters:** Create improvised filters using layers of cloth, sand, and charcoal to remove larger particles and improve water clarity.

3. **Chemical Treatment**

   - **Water Purification Tablets:** Add chemical tablets (chlorine dioxide, iodine) to untreated water to kill pathogens. Follow manufacturer instructions for dosage and contact time.

   - **Liquid Chlorine Bleach:** Use unscented liquid chlorine bleach (containing 5.25-6% sodium hypochlorite) to disinfect water. Add precise amounts per gallon and allow 30 minutes for disinfection.

4. **UV Purification**

   ○ **UV Sterilization Devices:** Use UV purifiers designed for outdoor use to kill bacteria, viruses, and protozoa in water. Ensure batteries are charged and devices are used according to manufacturer guidelines.

Water Conservation and Management

Optimize water use and storage to ensure long-term availability and sustainability in survival scenarios.

1. **Hydration Needs**

   ○ **Drink Regularly:** Consume water at regular intervals to prevent dehydration and maintain bodily functions.

   ○ **Monitor Output:** Pay attention to urine color and frequency as indicators of hydration status.

2. **Water Storage**

- o **Containers:** Use durable, lightweight containers for storing collected water. Seal tightly to prevent contamination.

- o **Cover and Shade:** Protect water containers from direct sunlight and debris to maintain water quality.

3. **Emergency Water Sources**

- o **Emergency Reserves:** Carry emergency water supplies or purification tools in your survival kit to ensure access to water in unforeseen circumstances.

- o **Responsible Use:** Conserve water by prioritizing essential needs and minimizing waste during survival situations.

Practical Exercises

1. **Water Sourcing:** Practice identifying and collecting water from different natural sources in your local environment.

2. **Purification Techniques:** Test various water purification methods (boiling, filtration, chemical treatment) on collected water. Evaluate effectiveness and taste.

3. **Emergency Scenarios:** Simulate emergency situations where water sources are limited. Practice water conservation and prioritize hydration needs.

Chapter 12: Wilderness First Aid and Medical Emergencies

In wilderness survival scenarios, being prepared to handle medical emergencies and provide basic first aid can be crucial for ensuring safety and increasing survival chances. This chapter covers essential wilderness first aid techniques, emergency preparedness, and strategies for managing injuries and medical conditions in remote environments.

Importance of Wilderness First Aid

Understanding wilderness first aid is critical for several reasons:

1. **Immediate Response:** Provides timely care to stabilize injuries and medical conditions until professional help is available.

2. **Prevention of Complications:** Reduces the risk of infection, shock, and further injury by addressing medical emergencies promptly.

3. **Promotion of Safety:** Enhances safety awareness and preparedness among individuals engaging in outdoor activities.

Basic First Aid Principles

Applying basic first aid principles ensures effective initial care in wilderness settings.

1. **Assessment and Prioritization**

   - **Primary Survey:** Assess the scene for safety hazards. Check the victim's responsiveness, airway, breathing, and circulation (ABCs).

   - **Secondary Survey:** Conduct a systematic head-to-toe assessment to identify injuries and medical conditions.

2. **Control Bleeding**

   - **Direct Pressure:** Apply direct pressure with a clean cloth or sterile dressing to control bleeding from wounds.

- **Elevation:** Raise the injured limb above heart level to slow bleeding, if possible.

- **Pressure Points:** Apply pressure to arterial pressure points to control severe bleeding not responsive to direct pressure.

3. **Manage Airway and Breathing**

- **Clear Airway:** Ensure the victim's airway is clear of obstructions. Perform the head-tilt, chin-lift maneuver if needed.

- **CPR:** Administer cardiopulmonary resuscitation (CPR) if the victim is unresponsive and not breathing normally.

4. **Treat Shock**

- **Lay Victim Down:** Place the victim on their back with legs elevated unless there is a head, leg, or spine injury.

- **Cover and Insulate:** Cover the victim with blankets or clothing to maintain body heat and prevent further shock.

Common Wilderness Injuries and Conditions

Recognizing and managing specific injuries and medical conditions encountered in the wilderness is essential.

1. **Traumatic Injuries**

   - **Fractures and Sprains:** Immobilize fractures and provide support using improvised splints and bandages.

   - **Burns:** Cool burns with clean water and protect with sterile dressings to prevent infection.

   - **Animal Bites and Stings:** Clean wounds thoroughly and monitor for signs of infection or allergic reactions.

2. **Environmental Injuries**

   - **Hypothermia:** Gradually warm the victim using dry clothing, blankets, and a heat source. Handle gently to prevent further heat loss.

○ **Heat Exhaustion and Heatstroke:** Move the victim to a cool, shaded area. Cool the body with water and fan to reduce body temperature.

3. **Medical Emergencies**

○ **Heart Attack:** Administer aspirin if available and monitor the victim's condition. Be prepared to perform CPR if necessary.

○ **Allergic Reactions:** Administer epinephrine (EpiPen) for severe allergic reactions (anaphylaxis). Monitor breathing and circulation.

Improvised Medical Techniques

Adaptation and improvisation are crucial when professional medical care and resources are unavailable.

1. **Improvised Splints and Bandages**

○ **Splints:** Use sticks, trekking poles, or rolled-up clothing to immobilize fractures and sprains.

- ○ **Bandages:** Use clean cloth, bandanas, or strips of clothing to secure dressings and create slings.

2. **Emergency Shelter and Comfort**

   - ○ **Insulation:** Use blankets, sleeping bags, or natural materials to provide insulation and warmth for injured or ill individuals.

   - ○ **Positioning:** Maintain a comfortable and stable position for victims to prevent exacerbation of injuries.

Communication and Rescue

Effectively communicating with emergency services and coordinating rescue efforts is vital for prompt evacuation and advanced medical care.

1. **Emergency Signaling**

   - ○ **Visual Signals:** Use mirrors, bright clothing, or signal fires to attract attention from rescuers.

- **Audible Signals:** Use whistles, horns, or shouting in intervals to signal distress.

2. **Emergency Contact Information**

   - **Emergency Plan:** Share trip details, routes, and expected return times with a trusted contact or emergency services.

   - **Communication Devices:** Carry communication devices such as satellite phones, Personal Locator Beacons (PLBs), or two-way radios for emergencies.

Practical Exercises

1. **Scenario Simulations:** Role-play wilderness first aid scenarios, practicing assessment, treatment, and evacuation procedures.

2. **First Aid Kits:** Assemble and familiarize yourself with contents of a wilderness first aid kit. Replenish supplies as needed.

3. **Team Exercises:** Collaborate with partners or groups to respond to simulated medical emergencies in outdoor settings.

Chapter 13: Mental and Psychological Preparedness

Surviving in the wilderness is not just about physical skills; mental and psychological resilience play a crucial role in overcoming challenges and maintaining morale. This chapter focuses on strategies for mental preparedness, stress management, and maintaining psychological well-being in wilderness survival situations.

Importance of Mental Preparedness

Maintaining a positive mental attitude and psychological resilience is vital for several reasons:

1. **Decision Making:** Clear thinking and rational decision-making under stress are essential for survival.

2. **Adaptability:** Flexibility and mental agility help adapt to changing conditions and unexpected challenges.

3. **Morale and Motivation:** Mental resilience boosts morale, motivation, and the will to survive.

Developing Mental Resilience

Building mental resilience involves cultivating certain attitudes and practices that enhance your ability to cope with adversity.

1. **Positive Mindset**

   o **Optimism:** Focus on solutions rather than problems. Believe in your ability to overcome challenges.

   o **Gratitude:** Acknowledge and appreciate small victories, resources, and support.

2. **Stress Management**

   o **Breathing Exercises:** Practice deep breathing and relaxation techniques to calm the mind and reduce stress.

- o **Mindfulness:** Stay present and aware of your surroundings. Practice mindfulness to manage anxiety and maintain focus.

3. **Adaptability**

- o **Flexibility:** Embrace uncertainty and adapt to changing circumstances. Be willing to adjust plans and expectations as needed.

- o **Problem-Solving:** Approach challenges with a systematic and creative problem-solving mindset.

Coping with Isolation and Loneliness

Isolation in wilderness settings can lead to feelings of loneliness and affect mental well-being. Strategies to manage isolation include:

1. **Routine and Structure**

    o **Daily Tasks:** Establish a routine for gathering food, maintaining shelter, and other essential tasks. Structure provides a sense of stability.

2. **Positive Distractions**

    o **Hobbies and Activities:** Engage in activities like journaling, drawing, or storytelling to occupy your mind and boost morale.

    o **Nature Connection:** Appreciate the beauty of nature. Take time to observe wildlife, sunsets, and natural phenomena.

3. **Social Connection**

    o **Self-Talk:** Maintain positive self-talk and encourage yourself during difficult moments.

    o **Imaginary Companionship:** Imagine conversations or interactions with loved ones or fictional characters to combat feelings of loneliness.

Dealing with Fear and Anxiety

Fear and anxiety are natural responses in survival situations. Techniques to manage fear include:

1. **Education and Preparation**

   - **Knowledge:** Educate yourself about wilderness survival techniques and potential risks. Preparedness reduces anxiety.

2. **Visualization and Mental Rehearsal**

   - **Visualize Success:** Mentally rehearse successful outcomes and visualize overcoming challenges to build confidence.

   - **Positive Affirmations:** Repeat positive affirmations or mantras to reinforce confidence and resilience.

3. **Grounding Techniques**

- **Focus on Senses:** Use sensory grounding techniques such as focusing on sights, sounds, and tactile sensations to stay present and calm.

- **Reality Check:** Challenge irrational thoughts and fears by assessing actual risks and immediate priorities.

Psychological First Aid

Providing psychological support to yourself and others in survival situations can enhance resilience and well-being.

1. **Active Listening**

   - **Empathetic Listening:** Listen actively and non-judgmentally to others' concerns and experiences.

   - **Validation:** Acknowledge feelings and emotions expressed by yourself and others.

2. **Encouragement and Support**

   - **Encouragement:** Offer words of encouragement and support to boost morale and motivation.

- Team Spirit: Foster camaraderie and teamwork among group members to share burdens and provide mutual support.

Practical Exercises

1. **Mindfulness Practice:** Engage in daily mindfulness meditation or relaxation exercises to enhance mental clarity and emotional stability.

2. **Solo Reflection:** Spend time alone in nature to reflect on personal strengths, goals, and sources of motivation.

3. **Role-Playing:** Role-play stressful scenarios and practice responding with calmness, rationality, and resilience.

Chapter 14: Shelter Building and Survival Shelters

Building effective shelters is essential for protection from the elements and ensuring comfort and safety in wilderness survival situations. This chapter explores various shelter types, construction techniques, and considerations for creating durable and functional shelters in diverse environmental conditions.

Importance of Shelter

Shelter serves critical purposes in wilderness survival:

1. **Protection from Elements:** Shields against rain, wind, sun, and temperature extremes to maintain body temperature and prevent hypothermia or hyperthermia.

2. **Safety and Security:** Provides a safe refuge from wildlife, insects, and potential hazards in the environment.

3. **Psychological Comfort:** Enhances morale, reduces stress, and promotes rest and recovery during challenging circumstances.

Types of Wilderness Shelters

Understanding different shelter types allows adaptation to varying terrain, weather conditions, and available resources.

1. **Debris Shelters**

   - **Lean-to:** Constructed by leaning branches or logs against a sturdy base, such as a fallen tree or rock wall. Cover with leaves, moss, or debris for insulation.

   - **A-Frame:** Uses two supports with a cross beam to create a steep, triangular roof. Covered with foliage, tarps, or other insulating materials.

   - **Dome or Wickiup:** Rounded structure using curved branches or saplings, often covered with grass, leaves, or bark for insulation.

2. **Tarp Shelters**

- Tarp Tent: Utilizes a lightweight tarp or poncho draped over a ridge line or between trees. Secured with cordage and stakes for stability.

- Plow Point: Similar to a tarp tent but with a low, triangular profile. Provides protection from wind and rain on one side.

3. Natural Shelters

- Caves or Rock Overhangs: Utilize natural rock formations for shelter, providing protection from weather and animals.

- Tree Wells or Hollows: Use hollowed-out tree trunks or large tree roots as natural shelters, providing insulation and protection.

Shelter Construction Techniques

Mastering shelter construction techniques ensures durability and functionality in various wilderness conditions.

1. **Site Selection**

   ○ **Terrain:** Choose flat or gently sloping ground free from rocks, roots, and standing water.

   ○ **Natural Features:** Utilize natural windbreaks, sun orientation, and drainage patterns for optimal shelter placement.

2. **Foundation and Support Structures**

   ○ **Base:** Clear ground and create a level foundation using rocks, logs, or compacted earth.

   ○ **Supports:** Use sturdy branches, saplings, or poles as framework supports for shelter structure.

3. **Insulation and Weatherproofing**

   ○ **Covering:** Layer shelter walls and roof with natural materials like leaves, pine needles, or grass for insulation and waterproofing.

- **Water Management:** Ensure proper drainage to prevent water accumulation inside the shelter during rain or melting snow.

Improvised and Emergency Shelters

Adaptation and improvisation are key when immediate shelter is necessary in survival situations.

1. **Emergency Shelter Techniques**

   - **Debris Huts:** Quickly assemble a framework of branches and cover with available debris and foliage.

   - **Poncho Shelter:** Use a poncho or emergency blanket draped over a sturdy rope or branch line. Secure edges with stakes or rocks.

2. **Snow Shelters**

   - **Snow Cave:** Dig into a snowbank to create an insulated shelter. Shape walls and ceiling for structural integrity and ventilation.

- **Quinzhee:** Build a mound of snow, allow it to settle, then hollow out the interior to create a dome-shaped shelter.

Shelter Maintenance and Upkeep

Regular maintenance ensures shelters remain functional and provide adequate protection over time.

1. **Repair and Reinforcement**

   - **Inspect regularly:** Check for damage, leaks, or structural weaknesses. Repair with available materials to maintain integrity.

   - **Reinforce:** Strengthen shelter walls and roof with additional layers of insulation or weatherproofing materials as needed.

2. **Sanitation and Hygiene**

   - **Cleanliness:** Keep shelter interior free from debris, insects, and moisture. Maintain a dry sleeping area to prevent dampness and mold.

- **Fire Safety:** Use caution with fires inside shelters. Ensure proper ventilation and clearance to prevent smoke inhalation and fire hazards.

Practical Exercises

1. **Shelter Building Drills:** Practice constructing different shelter types using natural and improvised materials.

2. **Overnight Shelters:** Spend a night in a self-built shelter to test durability, comfort, and protection against weather conditions.

3. **Emergency Scenarios:** Simulate scenarios requiring immediate shelter construction. Practice rapid deployment and adaptation to environmental challenges.

Chapter 15: Fire Craft and Fire Management

Fire is a vital tool in wilderness survival, providing warmth, light, protection, and the means to cook food and purify water. This chapter explores essential fire craft skills, techniques for fire starting and management, and safety considerations in various outdoor environments.

Importance of Fire in Survival

Understanding the importance of fire in wilderness survival is crucial for several reasons:

1. **Warmth and Comfort:** Provides heat in cold environments, helping to regulate body temperature and prevent hypothermia.

2. **Cooking and Food Preparation:** Enables cooking and preparation of wild edibles, improving nutritional intake and food safety.

3. **Signaling and Communication:** Acts as a visual and audible signal for rescuers or nearby individuals.

4. **Psychological Benefits:** Boosts morale, provides a sense of security, and fosters a connection with the natural environment.

Fire Starting Methods

Mastering various fire starting techniques ensures reliability and adaptability in different conditions.

1. **Primitive Methods**

   ○ **Friction Fire:** Use techniques such as the bow drill or hand drill to create fire by friction between wood components.

   ○ **Fire Plow:** Rub a stick along a groove in a softer wood base to generate heat and ignite tinder.

- **Flint and Steel:** Strike a flint or quartz rock against a steel striker to produce sparks, igniting char cloth or tinder.

2. **Modern Methods**

- **Fire Starters:** Use commercially available fire starters like ferrocerium rods (firesteel), magnesium blocks, or waterproof matches.

- **Lighters:** Carry reliable waterproof lighters for quick and efficient fire starting in various weather conditions.

3. **Improvised Methods**

- **Battery and Steel Wool:** Touch steel wool with the terminals of a battery to generate sparks and ignite tinder.

- **Solar Ignition:** Use a magnifying glass or convex lens to focus sunlight onto tinder for ignition.

Fire Lay and Structure

Understanding different fire lays enhances efficiency, control, and effectiveness in managing fires.

1. **Teepee Fire Lay**

   o **Structure:** Arrange kindling and firewood in a cone or teepee shape around a central tinder bundle.

   o **Advantages:** Promotes good airflow and rapid ignition, suitable for quickly building up a strong fire.

2. **Log Cabin Fire Lay**

   o **Structure:** Stack alternating layers of firewood in a square or log cabin pattern around a central tinder bundle.

   o **Advantages:** Creates a stable base with reduced need for frequent adjustment, ideal for longer-lasting fires and cooking.

3. **Lean-to Fire Lay**

- **Structure:** Lean larger fuel logs against a supporting log or rock wall, leaving space for tinder and kindling underneath.

- **Advantages:** Provides a reflective surface for heat and shelter from wind, suitable for windy conditions.

Fire Management and Safety

Practicing fire safety and responsible fire management minimizes risks and environmental impact.

1. **Site Selection**

   - **Clear Area:** Clear combustible materials and vegetation from the fire site, creating a fire-safe zone.

   - **Surface:** Choose bare soil or non-flammable surfaces for fire lay to prevent ground fires.

2. **Building and Maintaining Fires**

   - **Fuel Preparation:** Gather and prepare fuel in advance, organizing by size for efficient feeding into the fire.

- **Feeding and Tending:** Gradually add fuel to maintain a steady flame. Avoid smothering or overloading the fire with fuel.

3. **Extinguishing Fires**

   - **Douse with Water:** Pour water over the fire and stir thoroughly to extinguish embers and hot spots.

   - **Cover and Smother:** Cover the fire with dirt, sand, or ashes and stir to smother remaining embers.

   - **Monitor and Disperse:** Monitor the fire site for several hours after extinguishing to ensure no re-ignition occurs.

Fire in Survival Scenarios

Understanding the role of fire in specific survival scenarios enhances preparedness and decision-making.

1. **Emergency Signaling**

- Smoke Signals: Generate dense smoke by adding green vegetation or damp materials to the fire for signaling distress.

2. **Cooking and Food Preparation**

- Fire Pit Cooking: Use rocks or a dug-out fire pit to contain and control cooking fires for safe food preparation.

- Boiling Water: Purify water by bringing it to a rolling boil over a controlled fire to kill pathogens and make it safe for drinking.

Practical Exercises

1. **Fire Starting Challenges:** Practice various fire starting methods in different weather conditions (dry, wet, windy).

2. **Fire Lay Construction:** Build and maintain different fire lay structures to understand their advantages and adaptability.

3. **Fire Safety Drills:** Conduct fire safety drills, including site selection, fire management, and proper extinguishing techniques.

Chapter 16: Navigation and Orienteering

Navigation skills are essential for finding your way in the wilderness, whether you're exploring, hiking, or in a survival situation. This chapter covers fundamental techniques, tools, and strategies for effective navigation and orienteering in diverse outdoor environments.

Importance of Navigation Skills

Mastering navigation skills is crucial for several reasons:

1. **Safety and Risk Management:** Helps prevent getting lost and facilitates timely rescue in emergency situations.

2. **Route Planning:** Enables efficient travel by identifying key landmarks, terrain features, and water sources.

3. **Self-Sufficiency:** Reduces reliance on electronic devices and enhances self-reliance in remote areas.

Understanding Terrain and Topography

Understanding terrain and topography aids in route planning and navigation accuracy.

1. **Topographic Maps**

   o **Features:** Identify contour lines, elevation changes, water sources, and man-made structures.

   o **Scale and Legend:** Interpret map scale and legend to understand distances and symbols.

2. **Terrain Assessment**

   o **Natural Landmarks:** Recognize distinctive features such as mountains, valleys, rivers, and prominent rock formations.

   o **Vegetation and Soil Types:** Note vegetation density, soil composition, and ground conditions that affect travel.

Navigation Tools and Equipment

Utilizing appropriate tools enhances navigation accuracy and efficiency.

1. **Compass**

   ○ **Components:** Understand compass parts including magnetic needle, housing, and orienting arrow.

   ○ **Orientation:** Use compass to orient map and determine direction of travel (bearing).

2. **GPS Devices**

   ○ **Functionality:** Utilize GPS for accurate positioning, waypoint marking, and route tracking.

   ○ **Backup Power:** Carry spare batteries or rechargeable power sources for extended use.

3. **Natural Navigation**

   ○ **Sun and Stars:** Use sun's position and shadow lengths for direction (solar navigation).

- **North Star:** Locate Polaris (North Star) for nighttime navigation in the Northern Hemisphere.

Navigation Techniques

Employing effective navigation techniques ensures accurate direction finding and route following.

1. **Dead Reckoning**

    - **Pacing:** Measure distance by counting steps or using predetermined pace count.

    - **Handrailing:** Follow a linear terrain feature (e.g., river, ridge) as a guide to reach destination.

2. **Aiming Off**

    - **Offset Navigation:** Purposefully navigate slightly to the side of target, using linear feature to guide approach.

3. **Terrain Association**

- o **Relate Map to Terrain:** Match map features with observed terrain landmarks for precise location awareness.

Route Planning and Execution

Plan routes to optimize travel efficiency and safety in wilderness environments.

1. **Identify Waypoints**

   - o **Checkpoints:** Mark significant landmarks or waypoints along route for navigation verification.

   - o **Water Sources:** Plan routes near reliable water sources for hydration and resource access.

2. **Risk Assessment**

   - o **Hazards:** Identify potential hazards (steep terrain, water crossings, dense vegetation) along planned route.

   - o **Contingency Plans:** Develop alternative routes and emergency response plans for unexpected challenges.

Emergency Navigation Techniques

Prepare for situations where conventional navigation methods may not be available or practical.

1. **Map and Compass Skills**

   o **Map Only Navigation:** Use map features and terrain association without compass for direction finding.

   o **Shadow Stick Method:** Use shadow cast by stick or watch to estimate cardinal directions.

2. **Signaling for Help**

   o **Signal Fires:** Create visible smoke or flames during daylight for aerial search visibility.

   o **Ground Signals:** Use rocks, logs, or markers to create symbols or messages visible from air or ground.

Practical Exercises

1. **Map Reading:** Practice interpreting topographic maps and identifying terrain features.

2. **Compass Skills:** Conduct exercises to orient map, determine bearings, and navigate using compass.

3. **Field Navigation:** Navigate predefined routes or create navigation challenges in varied terrain and weather conditions.

Chapter 17: Foraging and Wild Edible Plants

Foraging for wild edible plants is a valuable skill in wilderness survival, providing essential nutrition, hydration, and medicinal benefits. This chapter explores the identification, harvesting, and preparation of wild edibles, emphasizing safety and sustainability in gathering food from natural environments.

Importance of Foraging for Wild Edibles

Foraging offers several benefits in survival scenarios and outdoor adventures:

1. **Nutritional Diversity:** Supplements diet with vitamins, minerals, and essential nutrients not found in processed foods.

2. **Hydration Source:** Identifies water-rich plants for hydration when clean water sources are scarce.

3. **Medicinal Uses:** Recognizes plants with medicinal properties for treating minor ailments and injuries.

Plant Identification and Safety

Accurate plant identification and safety considerations are crucial to avoid toxic or harmful species.

1. **Identification Methods**

   - **Field Guides:** Use botanical field guides with color photos, descriptions, and identification keys.

   - **Local Knowledge:** Learn from experienced foragers or indigenous communities familiar with regional flora.

2. **Safety Precautions**

   - **Avoidance:** Avoid plants with unfamiliar characteristics, strong odors, or bitter tastes that indicate potential toxicity.

   - **Universal Edibility Test:** Conduct a cautious test by first touching to lips, then chewing a small amount, and finally ingesting in small quantities.

Common Edible Plants and Their Uses

Explore edible plants commonly found in various ecosystems and their culinary and medicinal uses.

1. **Leafy Greens and Herbs**

   - **Dandelion:** Young leaves can be eaten raw or cooked, rich in vitamins A and C.

   - **Plantain:** Leaves are edible raw or cooked, known for soothing properties on insect bites and minor burns.

   - **Stinging Nettle:** Edible when cooked, rich in iron and vitamins A and C.

2. **Berries and Fruits**

   - **Wild Strawberries:** Small, sweet berries rich in vitamin C, eaten raw or added to desserts.

   - **Blackberries:** Sweet-tart berries high in antioxidants, used in jams, pies, or eaten fresh.

- Elderberries: Dark purple berries used in syrups and teas, known for immune-boosting properties.

3. **Roots and Tubers**

   - **Wild Carrot (Queen Anne's Lace):** Edible root when young, resembling domestic carrots.

   - **Burdock:** Edible root rich in fiber, often boiled or stir-fried as a vegetable.

   - **Wild Potato (Jerusalem Artichoke):** Tubers are edible raw or cooked, resembling the taste of potatoes.

Harvesting and Preparation Techniques

Proper harvesting and preparation methods ensure safety and nutritional benefits of wild edibles.

1. **Ethical Harvesting**

   - **Sustainability:** Harvest plants in small quantities, leaving enough for wildlife and future growth.

- Legal Considerations: Follow regulations regarding foraging on public lands and protected areas.

2. **Cleaning and Processing**

   - **Washing:** Rinse wild edibles thoroughly to remove dirt, insects, and contaminants.

   - **Cooking:** Boil, steam, or sauté wild plants to enhance flavor and neutralize potential toxins.

3. **Preservation Methods**

   - **Drying:** Air-dry or use a dehydrator to preserve herbs, flowers, and fruits for long-term storage.

   - **Canning and Pickling:** Preserve berries and vegetables in vinegar or brine for extended shelf life.

Medicinal and Practical Uses

Explore medicinal properties and practical applications of wild edibles for health and wellness.

1. **Medicinal Plants**

- o **Mullein:** Leaves and flowers used in teas or poultices for respiratory ailments and skin conditions.

- o **Yarrow:** Flowers and leaves brewed into teas for fever reduction and wound healing.

- o **Chickweed:** Edible plant used topically for soothing skin irritations and minor cuts.

2. **Survival Uses**

- o **Emergency Food:** Identify high-calorie plants like cattails (Typha) for emergency food sources.

- o **Tea and Infusions:** Brew teas from pine needles or mint for hydration and digestive aid.

Practical Exercises

1. **Plant Identification Walks:** Conduct guided walks to practice identifying and discussing wild edibles in different seasons.

2. **Foraging Expeditions:** Organize foraging trips to gather, identify, and prepare wild edibles under supervision.

3. **Wilderness Cooking:** Prepare meals using harvested wild edibles, incorporating them into recipes for nutritional diversity.

Made in United States
Troutdale, OR
07/16/2024

21267485R00084